If you purchase this calendar without its cover, it may be stolen. Neither the publisher nor the author is obligated to provide professional services in any way, legal, health, or in any form related to this book, its contents, advice, or otherwise.

The laws and practices vary from country to country and state to state.

If legal or professional information is required, the purchaser or the reader should seek it privately and in a manner best suited to their particular needs and circumstances.

The author and publisher expressly disclaim any liability that may be incurred from the information within this book.

All rights reserved. No part of this book, including the interior design, images, cover design, diagrams, or any intellectual property (IP), icons, and photographs, may be reproduced or transmitted in any form by any means (electronic, photocopying, recording, or otherwise) without the prior permission of the publisher. ©

Copyright© 2024 MSI Australia
All rights reserved.
ISBN: 978-1-7636806-3-0

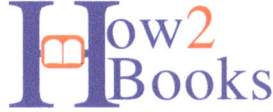

Published by How2Books
Under license from MSI Ltd, Australia
Company Registration No: 96963518255
NSW, Australia

See our website: www.how2books.com.au
Or contact by email: sales@how2books.com.au
Covers and Copyright owned by MSI, Australia
MSI acknowledges the author and images, text, and photographs used in this book.

10% of each book's sale helps support Diabetes Type One and Cancer Research.

YOUR NOTES

YOUR NOTES

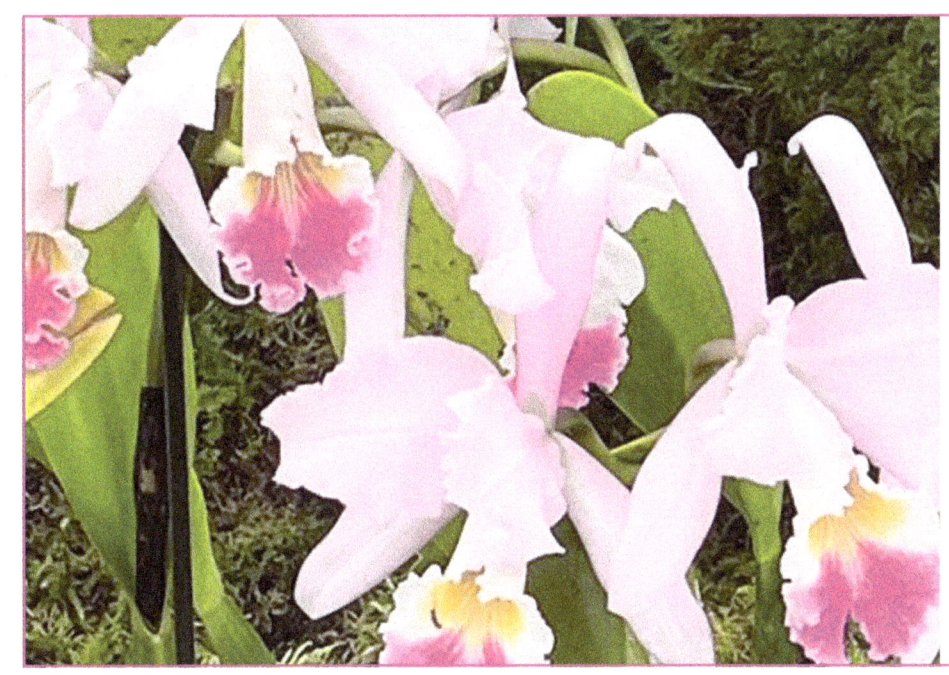

Beautiful cattleya orchids, rich in colour, shape, and presentation.

JANUARY

Monday	Tuesday	Wednesday	Thursday	Friday	Saturday	Sunday
		1	2	3	4	5
6	7	8	9	10	11	12
13	14	15	16	17	18	19
20	21	22	23	24	25	26
27	28	29	30	31		

YOUR NOTES

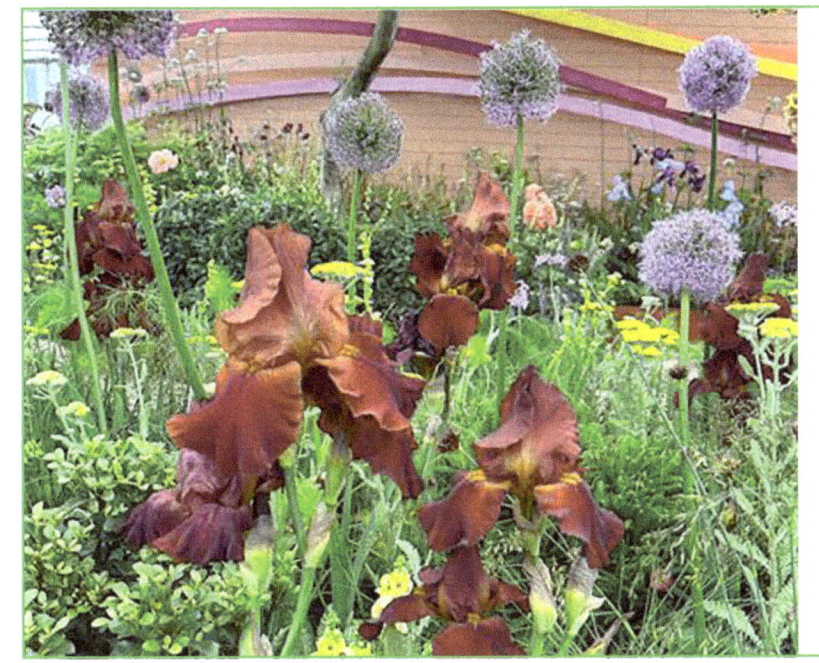

Just one of the many natural gardens on display at Chelsea this year. With true natural and true plantings encouraged, the combinations of colours and combinations are refreshing and a pleasure to see...

FEBRUARY

Monday	Tuesday	Wednesday	Thursday	Friday	Saturday	Sunday
					1	2
3	4	5	6	7	8	9
10	11	12	13	14	15	16
17	18	19	20	21	22	23
24	25	26	27	28		

YOUR NOTES

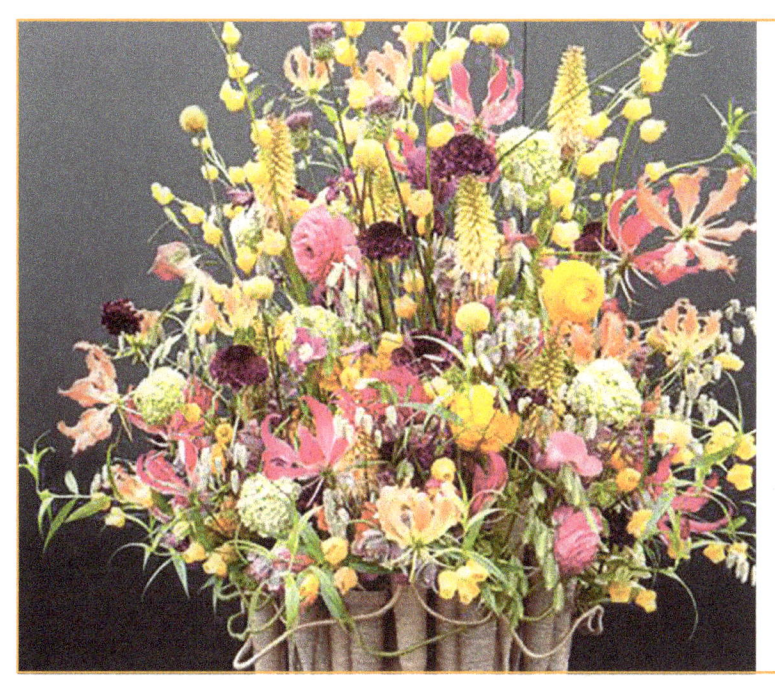

Floral artists and florists are now seeking alternative and creative ideas to create different but striking floral presentations and arrangements.

MARCH

Monday	Tuesday	Wednesday	Thursday	Friday	Saturday	Sunday
					1	2
3	4	5	6	7	8	9
10	11	12	13	14	15	16
17	18	19	20	21	22	23
24	25	26	27	28	29	30
31						

YOUR NOTES

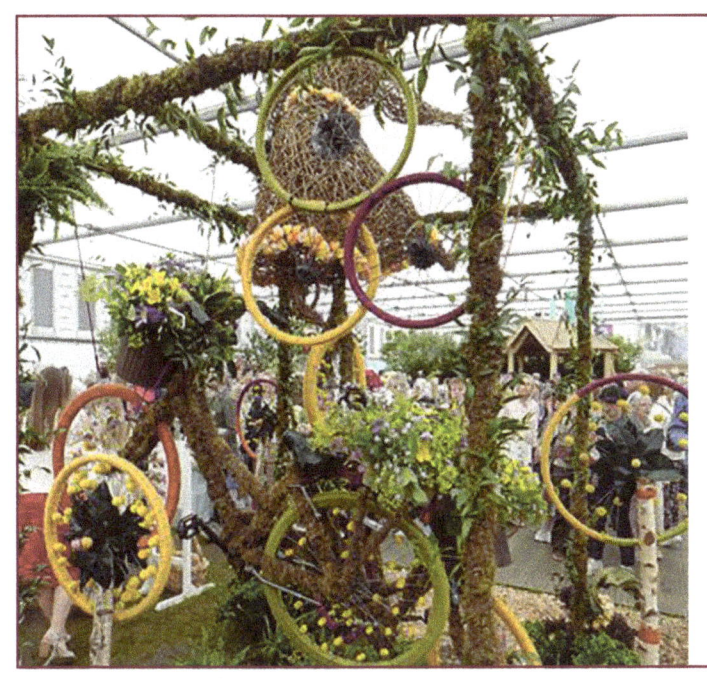

When the human imagination is allowed to think Outside the Box it is amazing to see what creativity comes forth, and through ingenuity, a story is told...!

APRIL

Monday	Tuesday	Wednesday	Thursday	Friday	Saturday	Sunday
	1	2	3	4	5	6
7	8	9	10	11	12	13
14	15	16	17	18	19	20
21	22	23	24	25	26	27
28	29	30				

YOUR NOTES

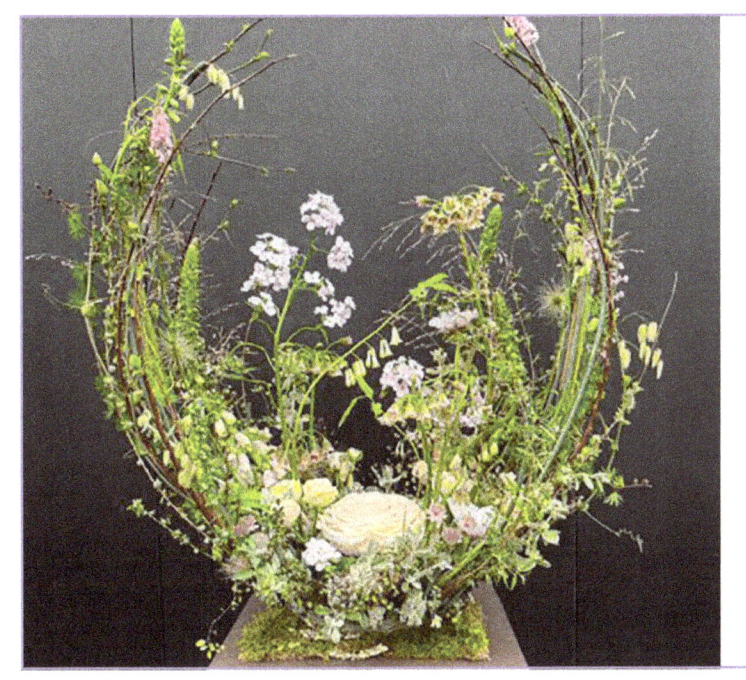

The opposite shows a truly beautiful arrangement. Though a traditional line arrangement is seen, the placements are loose and delicate... The anchor point is the large full-blown rose at the middle and focal point of the design.

MAY

Monday	Tuesday	Wednesday	Thursday	Friday	Saturday	Sunday
			1	2	3	4
5	6	7	8	9	10	11
12	13	14	15	16	17	18
19	20	21	22	23	24	25
26	27	28	29	30	31	

YOUR NOTES

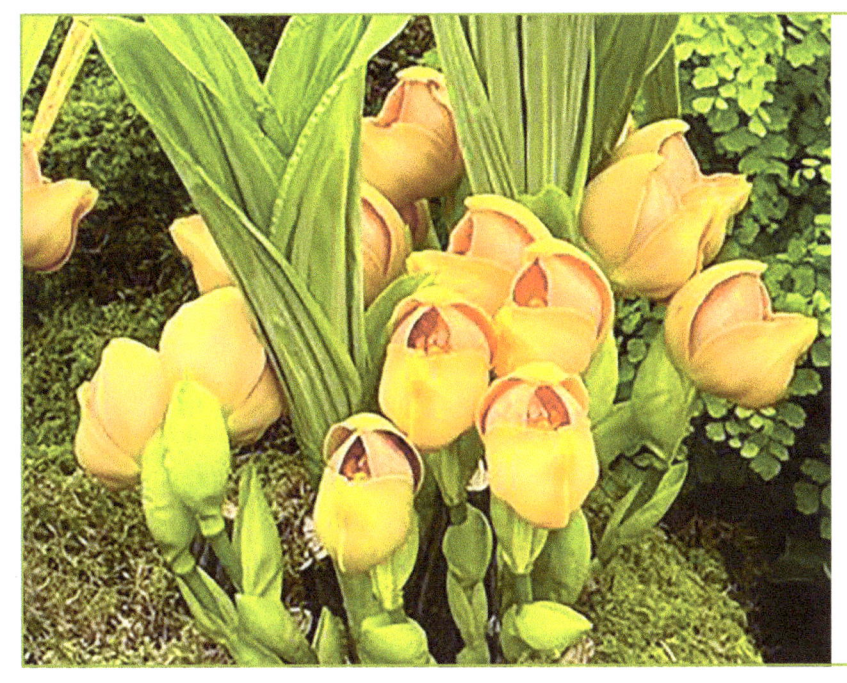

Swaddle Baby orchids seen in the opposite photograph are unique and ancient flowers that are truly mesmerizing and fascinating...

JUNE

Monday	Tuesday	Wednesday	Thursday	Friday	Saturday	Sunday
						1
2	3	4	5	6	7	8
9	10	11	12	13	14	15
16	17	18	19	20	21	22
23	24	25	26	27	28	29
30						

YOUR NOTES

YOUR NOTES

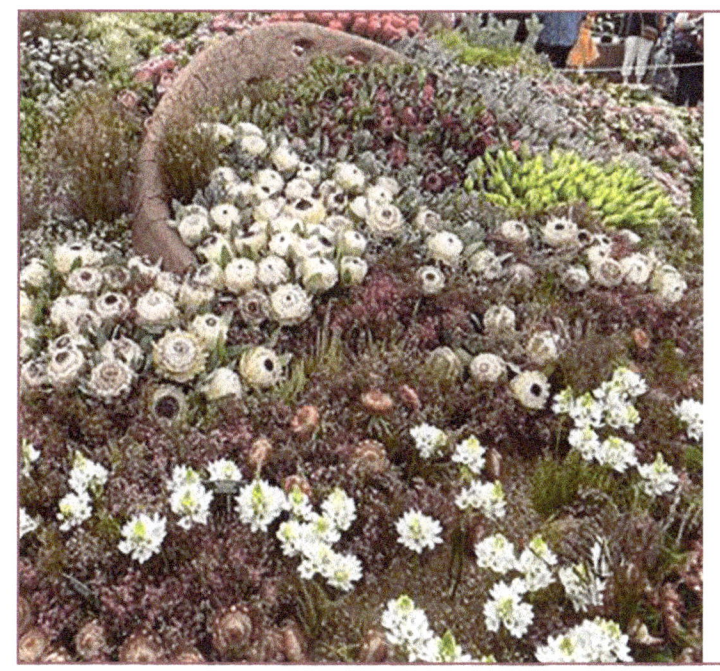

A display featuring many different types of proteas. The extent of the stand was vast with many incredible plantings thus, creating an explosion of colour... It was difficult not to be over-awed by the magnificence of the effort, time, and dedication to such a beautiful native and national flower of South Africa.

JULY

Monday	Tuesday	Wednesday	Thursday	Friday	Saturday	Sunday
	1	2	3	4	5	6
7	8	9	10	11	12	13
14	15	16	17	18	19	20
21	22	23	24	25	26	27
28	29	30	31			

YOUR NOTES

YOUR NOTES

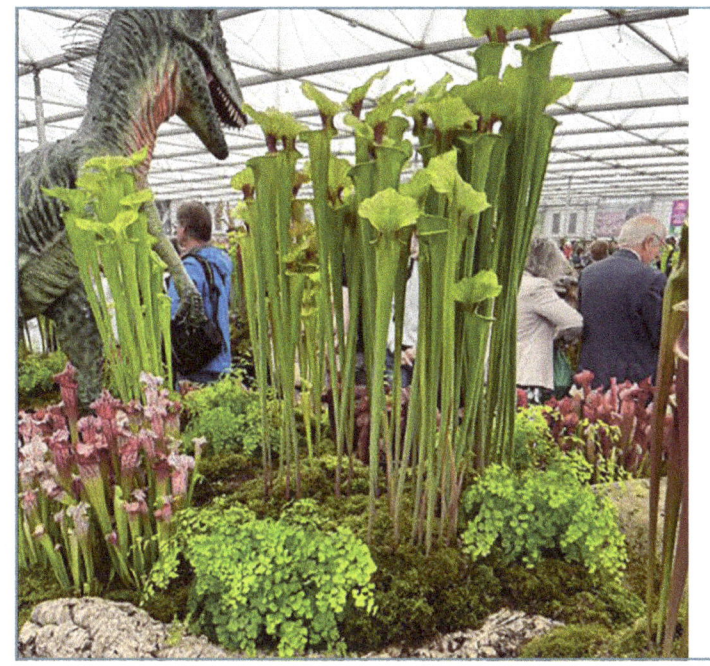

Sarracenias were seen in a range of different colours, some were by identity, shorter varieties as seen in the red, and then the tall green, which became elegant and a 'show stopper...!'

AUGUST

Monday	Tuesday	Wednesday	Thursday	Friday	Saturday	Sunday
				1	2	3
4	5	6	7	8	9	10
11	12	13	14	15	16	17
18	19	20	21	22	23	24
25	26	27	28	29	30	31

YOUR NOTES

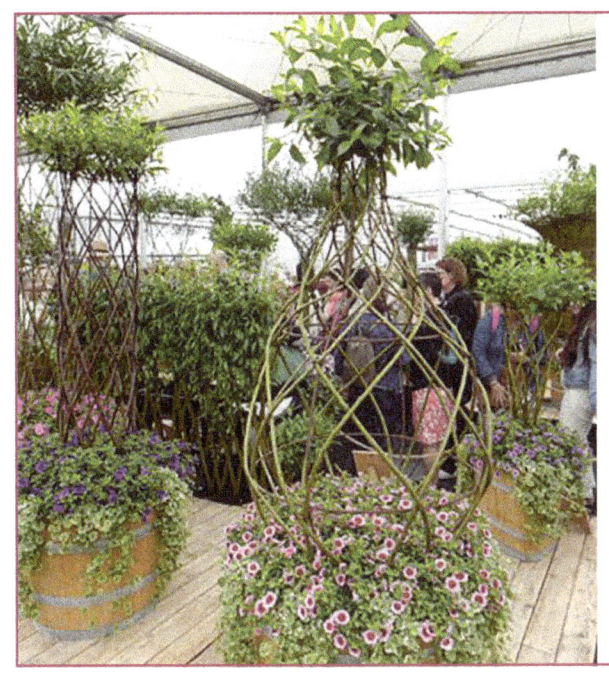

*Art expression is always interesting.
In the opposite, it can be seen how growing
plants are used as part of the visual display
creating voids, space and motion...*

SEPTEMBER

Monday	Tuesday	Wednesday	Thursday	Friday	Saturday	Sunday
1	2	3	4	5	6	7
8	9	10	11	12	13	14
15	16	17	18	19	20	21
22	23	24	25	26	27	28
29	30					

YOUR NOTES

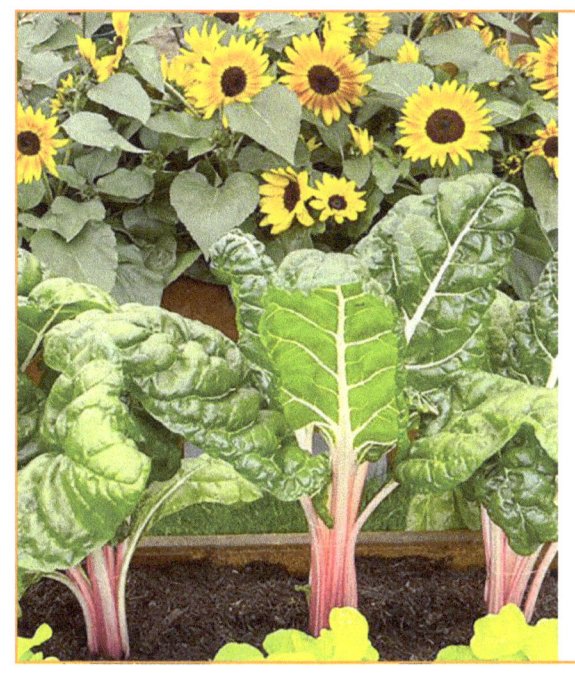

A striking display can be created through thought and imagination in any garden. In the opposite, the careful plantings of rhubarb and sunflowers create interest, different shapes and a pleasing presentation...

OCTOBER

Monday	Tuesday	Wednesday	Thursday	Friday	Saturday	Sunday
		1	2	3	4	5
6	7	8	9	10	11	12
13	14	15	16	17	18	19
20	21	22	23	24	25	26
27	28	29	30	31		

YOUR NOTES

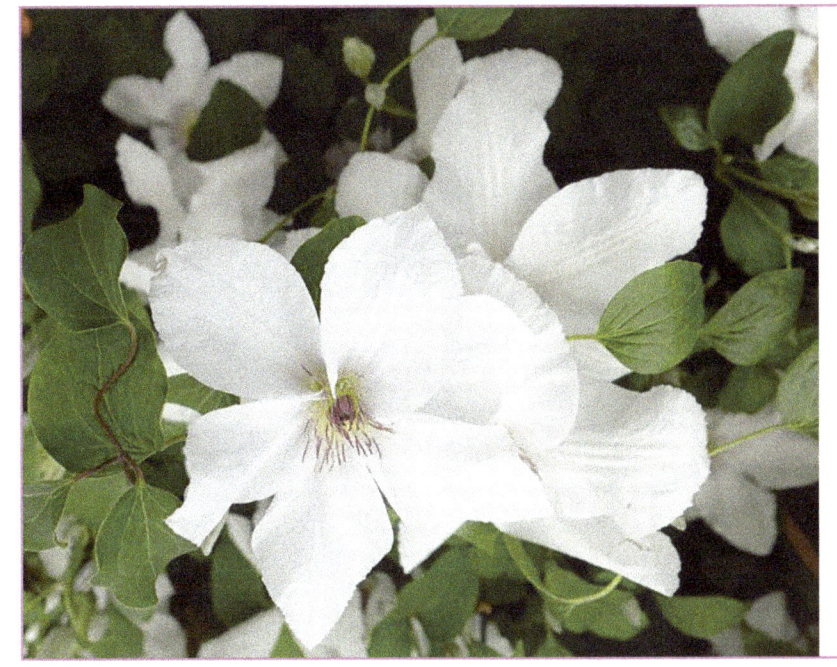

Such perfect white flowers are always difficult to resist, and here, the clematis shows off its beauty and the heavenly space it occupies. With a mass showing of these larger flowers than usually produced by the plant, the display was inspirational and beautiful to see...

NOVEMBER

Monday	Tuesday	Wednesday	Thursday	Friday	Saturday	Sunday
					1	2
3	4	5	6	7	8	9
10	11	12	13	14	15	16
17	18	19	20	21	22	23
24	25	26	27	28	29	30

YOUR NOTES

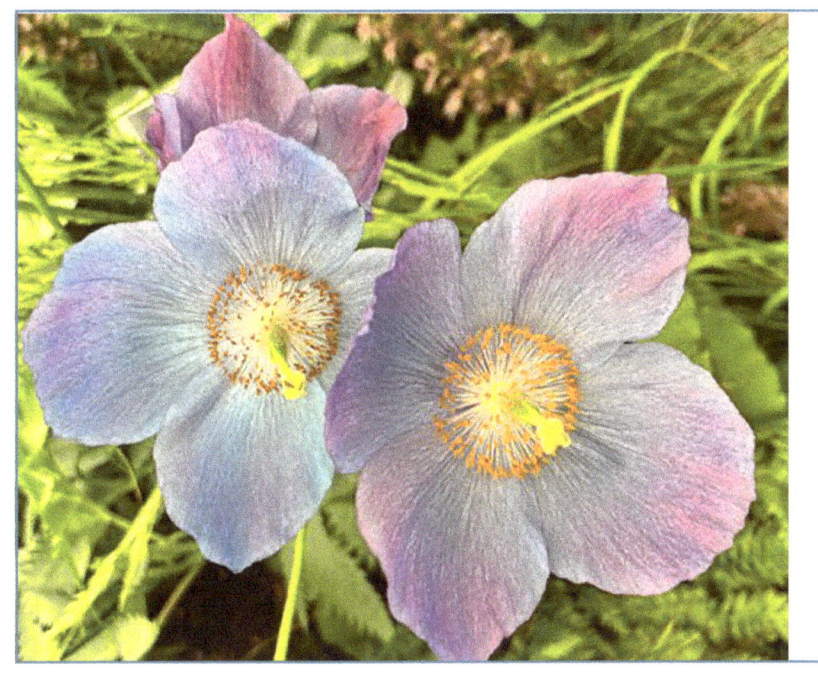

*By far, one of the most outstanding flowers seen at Chelsea in 2024 was the opposite Blue Poppy.
As can be seen, the variations from blues to different crimson tones and then the center of the flower reveal another amazing spectacle ...!
It isn't difficult to believe that nature can produce such visual delights...*

DECEMBER

Monday	Tuesday	Wednesday	Thursday	Friday	Saturday	Sunday
1	2	3	4	5	6	7
8	9	10	11	12	13	14
15	16	17	18	19	20	21
22	23	24	25	26	27	28
29	30	31				

YOUR NOTES

YOUR NOTES